PALEO DIET 101

PALEO DIET 101

WHAT IS THE PALEO DIET, PALEO DIET RECIPES AND CREATING A HEALTHY PALEO DIET

Miley Smith

Table of Content

Chapter 1 - Introduction

Living In A Fat And Unhealthy World

Look at the people around us. Many are facing a problem with obesity. This is because of a great eating problem which plaques many people have. With the rise of technology, education and healthcare; there are still many people who have yet to learn how to eat well.

For many of us, the problem is that we have is that we have a lifestyle which isn't optimal for existence and leaves the body with too many unwanted calories. Because of this, there is a great call to start eating based on the Paleo diet - a method of eating that goes with evolution.

In the past, the human body was trained to deal with food scarcity. That was before fatty and high calories foods were present. The problem is that, due to technology and the Agrarian revolution, it was possible to create an excess of food. As such, many people eat way too much. They eat out of boredom, loneliness and whenever negative emotions that they experience.

In the modern diet, we lack a balanced supply of macro and micronutrients. When the body is experiencing a lack of a type of nutrient, a hunger stimulus would be send to the brain and this causes you to eat more. However, it you don't eat the right form of food that produces these nutrients; you end up eating excessively but lacking of the nutrients of what you need. This becomes the major cause of obesity.

Besides overeating, eating wrongly is also a major cause of human obesity. Human beings have been eating unnatural foods for way too long. These are foods which have been heavily processed and artificial in nature. It doesn't just pile on the pounds but would also make the body at risk of many forms of diseases. This is a health risk in the modern bane of living. Natural food has lost it place to fast food.

Another problem that we face is the fact that we live in a sedentary lifestyle. This is a main problem of the modern lifestyle where we have very little exercise. Because of work stress, very little exercise time is afforded to individuals. Individuals don't have time for this simple act and it affects their health over the long term.

Many modern people have no idea how important exercise is. In the past, people have more time at their disposal. There was more time for leisure and life was less stressful. The human body was naturally fitter without needing to dedicate so much time for exercise. In the past when men were a food gatherer, the body was naturally fitter due to their constant movement to find for food.

Sedentary lifestyle isn't a problem that affects only adults but kids as well. Children in the modern generation are spending more time playing their computer games and staying indoors. This in turn results in obese children.

Although obesity can be a very serious problem, it could also be a symptom of other forms of diseases. Diseases like diabetes and other genetic problems could cause obesity. The individual might eat normally but put on a tremendous amount of weight. This is because any food that they eat would be converted to fat and they would gain a lot of weight. This is normally due to a problem in the genes.

It should also be known that obesity can cause a range of other diseases. This includes heart disease or diabetes. Unless the patient finds a real cure for their problem, the body would be headed for ruin.

It should be clear that obesity is a major problem and many people are looking to lose weight. The modern fitness diet would call for a limitation of calories to lose weight. This method would only be beneficial to a certain extent. You need to understand that without the proper supply of all the micro nutrients, the body would still be hungry. This causes you to break your diet and eat excessively.

You can succeed with a health fitness diet without the urge of binging by taking up the Paleo diet. The Paleo diet gets its philosophy from the fact that primitive people didn't eat any processed food but they were healthy. They are immune to many of the modern day diseases. This diet has went mainstream in 2005 when many celebrities started embracing this lifestyle. Many books and articles are written about this diet.

The Paleo diet includes eating unprocessed meat, fresh vegetables, fresh fruits and nuts. It is a diet which has a lot of fiber and would leave you feeling full without giving you an excessive amount of calories. This diet is low on oils and refined sugars. By eliminating these two ingredients, it creates a calorie deficit and a nutrient surplus which leads to a successful weight loss.

If any weight loss problem is to be successful implemented, it would have to be done based on evolutionary genetics. This suggests that we would need to replace our diets with those of our ancestors. It may be difficult for us to follow entirely; however, it is still possible to mimic it as closely as possible.

The History Of The Paleo Diet

The Paleo diet is based on an ancient diet that includes animals and other foods which were being consumed more than 2.5 million years ago during the Palaeolithic era. This diet is a gluten and preservative-free diet. It is focused on consuming certain type of food such as eggs, fish, vegetables, potatoes, roots, fruits, nuts and grass-fed pasture raised meats. In this sub-chapter, you would learn about the history of this diet.

This diet started out when a gastroenterologist by the name of Walter Voegtlin published a ground-breaking book that highlighted a modern version of the diet. He arrived at this conclusion after learning the eating habits of the people in the Palaeolithic age. He was looking for a cure for Crohn's disease, Irritable Bowel Syndrome and Colitis. From his research, he has found that those who followed such a Palaeolithic would be free from such diseases.

The version which he has shared in the book is based on the reasoning there isn't much human genetic changes since the Palaeolithic era. From his research, he has found that humans are supposed to eat primarily proteins and fats, while eating little carbohydrates.

In a few years later, Melvin Konner, an anthropologist learned the concepts of the Palaeolithic Diet. He wrote a paper with the assistance of his associate named Boyd Eaton. Their work got great publicity and from here, professionals in the medical field started discussing the diet that becomes an important part of Paleo diet history. Many doctors became convinced about the advantages of this diet.

A few years later, a book was written by the two of them again. They published a detailed information about the book but was written with a slight twist. Instead of focusing on food which shouldn't be included in the diet, they talked about why it is important to eat some portion of fats, proteins and carbohydrates according to the Palaeolithic era.

This is a slight change from the book written by Walter Voegtlin. In this diet, some food which weren't allowed by Voegtlin were allowed. It permitted agricultural foods such as brown rice, whole grain bread and other dairy products like skimmed milk. Their rationale was that the nutrient proportion and not the food choice was what made the Paleo Diet healthy.

In the 1990s, more nutritionists and doctors began to back this theory of starting with the Paleo Diet. Many doctors start recommending this diet to their patients and it becomes an integral part of a healthy eating plan for patients who were suffering from many diseases.

A great deal of them relied on the original concept where the food taken was before the introduction of agricultural. More and more people start to get drawn to this diet. It started to be accepted by more and more people. In the next sub-chapter, you would get a more detailed understanding about how the Paleo Diet works.

Paleo Diet Compared To Other Diets

If you are keen to lose weight, there are many options available. How would you know which of it works or don't? From the history of the Paleo Diet, it is certain that there are a great number of people who are using this program and getting quality results. It is a tested method that many people have found success with. This isn't a crash diet. You don't have to starve or go on a binding diet, which is often what other diets is based on.

When it comes to the Paleo Diet, there are several options but there are certain no-nos. Processed food is a definite NO as they aren't available to Palaeolithic people. As you develop the Paleo diet, you would stay healthy, build strength and lose weight. However, you wouldn't be able to build muscles mass. You would become leaner while not hurting your metabolic rate.

There is a huge problem with other forms of diets. Research has proven that when you go on a restricted diet for a week, the body enters into starvation mode. From this point, you would generally cheat by eating more of your favorite food, which is often unhealthy. You put your body in a bad position as you try to force the body to work against how it normally works.

Unlike other diet programs, the Paleo Diet works with the body. This program is essentially about what food you need to eat and what shouldn't be eaten. This would be discussed thoroughly in the next chapter. As you read the book, you would learn how to get rid of weight but also satisfy certain food cravings.

You would be able to lose weight permanently. Unlike other forms of dieting programs, you won't put on weight as it is more of a lifestyle change. You wouldn't harm your metabolism or lose any muscle mass. You wouldn't need to count calories while on this Paleo Diet nor punish yourself as the Paleo Diet recipes are extremely delicious. It doesn't even matter if obesity is in your genes. The Paleo Diet have helped many people who were genetically obese deal with their weight problem.

Another great thing about the Paleo Diet is that the effects can be seen in as little as two week. The moment the body starts with this diet, it puts itself in a detox process. It may be a tough first few days as it takes time for the body to get used to it. The diet of high nutrition fruits and vegetables, lean meats and eggs can be tough for someone who hasn't been eating well.

The key to being successful in the Paleo Diet is to eat healthy. Paleo diet weight loss programs would include detailed healthy food recipes that are easy to make but extremely delicious. You would learn about it in future chapters. You would also learn how to control yourself from frequent snacking and incessant food cravings.

Chapter 2 - How The Paleo Diet Works

The main reason why the Paleo Diet is so effective is due to its high nutritional content. The Paleo Diet helps to maintain your weight over a long period. This is partly due to the two forms of fiber in them - soluble and insoluble fiber.

Soluble fiber in the Paleo diet can be dissolved in water and upon dissolving, produces a gel like substance. This is helpful as it would trap the bad cholesterol particles like the low-density lipoprotein (LDL). This is important in preventing heart diseases from occurring due to the excessive accumulation of fat in the blood vessels. It has been proven that by following the Paleo diet for a short period, it could drastically reduce cholesterol accumulation.

Besides that, the gelatinous substance would change the properties of the digested food in the stomach. From this change, the content would move slowly and gives a feeling of fullness. This would ensure that the individual wouldn't eat excessively. It would also result in a more complete digestion activity by the enzymes.

These functions are also important in regulating the excessive nutrients in the blood. As soluble fiber prolongs digestion, there would be more time for nutrients to enter the blood stream without the body having to eat more food. It is very important for those with diabetics. As sugar molecules and carbohydrates would undergo a slower digestion due to soluble fiber, the body would have more time to convert such energy before the desire to eat arises again. As such, the pile up of sugar in the blood is reduced.

There are also benefits from the insoluble fiber taken. It helps to push the contents in the intestines. This is simply done by absorbing water and becoming heavier than the norm. This excess weight and expansion would exert more pressure in the Gastrointestinal (GI) tract and pushes the contents out of the body smoothly. As such, the bowel movement would be more regulated and constipation can be prevented.

Living a Paleo diet also helps to maintain the pH levels in the intestines. Generally, pH is an indicator of the acidity. If the stomach is too acidic, there is a higher chance of cancer. Paleo dieters would be able to reduce their acidic levels in their stomach. Besides that, a Paleo diet would also help reduce the risk of many other forms of cancer.

From the other chapters of this book, you would learn about the various food you eat from the Paleo diet. You would find that the natural carbohydrates found from the diet which is being recommended are very rich with energy. The energy would be released almost instantly and it has been proven to help individuals to enhance work performances within a mere half hour period.

One important part of the Paleo diet is the fact that you shouldn't take milk. This is something which surprises many people. Many people have been brought up to believe that milk is something nutritious and provides a balance nutrient.

Why You Shouldn't Take Milk And Alcohol

There are certain people who have an immune system reaction whenever they consume milk. The main cause is due to the proteins which are present in the milk. Certain people have an immune system that couldn't adapt to such proteins and would consider proteins in their foreign bodies.

As such, when these people take milk, their immune system would rush to counter and flush them out of the body. This causes a food allergic reaction. It should be clear that having a milk allergy is completely different with having lactose intolerance. Lactose intolerance is simply a delayed reaction to a certain food protein. This isn't an allergic reaction and couldn't be detected by an allergy test. However, both the symptoms seem the same to the common laymen.

It should be clear that the Paleo diet doesn't recommend taking milk from other animals. This is because most of the milk that you buy from the store are simply processed products. Like said from the previous chapter, you shouldn't take any processed food when on the Paleo diet.

Milk and other dairy products are a main cause of many healthy related issues like cardiovascular disease. Because of their processing, the naturalness is lost. As such, if you are following the Paleo diet, you shouldn't take any dairy products.

Another aspect of the Paleo diet is to ensure that you don't indulge in alcohol. It is already well known when it comes to the dangers of alcohol. Alcohol is an intoxicant and excessive consumption would make the body work harder to get rid of it.

Taking excessive amount of alcohol would cause a violent reaction. The person would also lose muscle control, lose strength and would affect in a slurred speaking condition.

Why You Need To Avoid Grains

In the past few years, grains have become an issue of controversy in the nutrition world. Americans are extremely affected because they consume a great amount of grain, either directly or indirectly. Grains are eaten in the form of cereal, pasta, bread and other baked products. It is also a main ingredient in processed foods.

Grains are essentially the main meal for many animals. This is especially so for animals raised for meat such as cows and chickens. As such, it is important to think about the effects of grains on our health and environment.

Many people believe that eating grains is important to getting your source of fiber. To avoid constipation, it is better to get your fiber from vegetables and fruits. Fiber from grains would actually irritate the digestive system. Besides that, you can also get other important vitamins and minerals from other foods.

The thing for many people is that advertisements on the TV tell that whole grains are good for you. This is normally a misinformation told by the companies selling the products. They might mention a research or so on, but most of the time the claims have been paid for by themselves.

If you want to give up grain, then the first thing you need to do is to consider whether if you are addicted to eating them. One of the best guides to learn about grains and losing weight quickly is the **Paleo Burn System**.

When I started to ditch grains, I felt terrible for a few weeks. I remember feeling a sense of headache and tiredness. It was a real test of my willpower but by the time your body is used to it, you would be able to feel much better and lose weight. You could also read about how this guy managed to help all his family members lose more than 30 pounds.

Check it out now at:-

paleoburn.paleodiet101.info

Nutrients From The Paleo Diet

By going on the Paleo diet, you would be able to focus on eating a great deal of nutrients that you would normally miss in a normal diet. One of them is Vitamin A. This vitamin is known as an anti-oxidant and helps prevent cells from the possible harmful effect of oxygen.

Oxygen, despite being essential to living, can be very harmful towards your biology. The Paleo diet is filled with anti-oxidants and together with other vitamins, it helps neutralize free radicals. Free radicals are something that would radicalize the healthy cells in your body and damage them.

When there are anti-oxidants in your body, it would help to make your skin healthy and blemish free. This would reduce the aging of your skin and helps prevent night-blindness. Vitamin A is also helpful in strengthening your bones and helps prevent certain respiratory diseases.

Another great benefit of the Paleo diet is that it helps improve clotting properties of your blood in those affected by hemophilia. Those women who suffer from excessive menstrual bleeding would also benefit tremendously from this diet because it is known as a holistic diet. There have been many cases of women who have suffered from such a diet and took on the Paleo diet. They have reported that it helps to normalize the menstrual cycle and makes the bleeding normal. Women who suffer from osteoporosis could also benefit from this diet as their bones would be strengthened.

Another great source of anti-oxidants is found in Vitamin C. This nutrient would help to maintain the structure and elasticity of blood vessels. For the blood to flow properly, it has to be maintained at its proper shape. This would also help to prevent undue stress on the heart and maintain the heart muscle itself.

The Paleo diet helps to protect the body from sun burns. This is because the Paleo diet is filled with Vitamin E and this helps to prevent the skin from damage of ultra violet rays of the sun. It would also provide against certain skin diseases like skin allergic inflammation and psoriasis.

Potassium, calcium and magnesium are three minerals which would help the body regular blood flow and control pressure in the small capillaries. It has been reported when people with high blood pressure start consuming Paleo foods, their blood pressure would start to decrease.

Paleo Helps You Lose Weight Naturally

The problem with most weight loss programs is that they focus on starving or exercising too much. This works against the natural tendencies of the human body. That is the reason why many people have tried many different weight loss programs but seems to have no results. They might lose a bit of weight and then put it on back after some time.

That is where the Paleo diet becomes so successful. The Paleo diet is a diet program which works with the body's natural tendencies. There isn't any calorie count or crash diet. Crash diet programs suggest that it you force the body to reduce the calories intake, you would lose weight over time. However, you would definitely gain it back the moment you stop that diet.

As such, the only solution is to eat healthy. The Paleo diet is indeed a revolution in the process of losing weight. You wouldn't need to starve or refrain from your favorite food but could still lose a tremendous amount of weight. For you to succeed in this diet, you would have to understand how your body works.

The logic is simple. When you make your body starve, your metabolism would shut down to conserve the resources. When such a thing happens, the fat you eat wouldn't get burn properly. Don't worry if your family members have obesity in the genes. As said before, the Paleo diet could help you drastically lose weight regardless of your genes.

Why You Shouldn't Starve

I have shared the power that the Paleo diet has when it comes to losing weight. Because it doesn't involve starving, it works better with the body's natural tendencies. Starving to lose weight can create certain other health problems like acid reflux or GERD. Acid reflux is a problem that could happen to anyone and could be chronic or acute. For many people, it can be very uncomfortable and the symptoms can last for a few years.

Eating the Paleo diet would give you a grip on the problem that you have. You would better understand the causes of your problem. You would also understand why modern medicine remedies haven't worked for you. It is also important to understand this relationship between diet, acid reflux and physical exercise. It may seem absurd, but you would learn about it in more detailed.

Those who suffer from diabetes should be on the Paleo diet. Those who are suffering from diabetics cannot go on crash diet programs which induce starvation. By taking on a Paleo diet, this would help the diabetic fight off this condition.

By eating a natural diet, it would be very beneficial in keeping the body clean and helps to detox it by itself. From this later chapters in the book, you would learn about the best combination to ensure that your body is healthy. By following the Paleo diet, you would be amazed to know that there is an incredible amount of acid in your body. Those who have utilize these diet would be able to get rid from many long standing health conditions that are acidic-based.

General Benefits Of Paleo Diet

From the past few years, the Paleo diet has become popular mainly because of its various health benefits. If you are considering going on this diet yourself, these are certain health benefits that you should consider. They include:

1. **Lose Weight Quickly** - I have explained how you can lose weight. The process of losing weight is difficult for many people because they look to go on crazy diets or eating foods which aren't good for them. It should be clear from the explanation in the previous sub-chapters.

2. **Great Energy** - Many people feel tired and lethargic after eating a big meal full of carbohydrates and fats. Many meals would make you feel terrible because they don't have any good nutrition for your daily needs. As you change the food you eat to healthy food, you would have more energy and feel great.

3. **More Nutritious** - It is hard to get proper nutrition when you are eating a diet of junk food, candies and fast food. Eating Paleo food ensures that you would get many essential nutrients. The food you eat would be filled with fiber, vitamins and other nutrients. They are great for your body.

4. **Deal Better With Allergy** - When dealing with allergies, the cause of many of them is the food you eat. Junk food causes many sorts of allergies because they are heavily

processed. Eating healthier food from the Paleo diet ensures that you don't have to worry about food allergens.

5. **Easy To Cook** - Although I didn't explain the process of cooking in the book, I can tell you that cooking Paleo food is very easy. You can find many different recipes through the resources in this book and they all taste great as well. As such, it makes it much easier to eat healthy.

These benefits are certainly things you should consider if you want to switch to a Paleo diet permanently.

What To Eat And Avoid

I have gone into detailed about the benefits of the Paleo diet. In order to follow the Paleo diet effectively, there are certain food that you should take and some you should avoid.

Among the food you should eat include:

- **Fruits** - Fruits such as apples and oranges are great for the Paleo diet. However, like anything else, you should always take them in moderation. You should also make sure that you don't consume dried fruits as they are normally processed. Other fruits such as bananas and grapes should be avoided because they contain a high amount of sugar.
- **Vegetables** - This is perhaps the most important part of the Paleo diet. Vegetables are an important part of people in the Palaeolithic era. However, it should be noted that consuming starchy vegetables like sweet potatoes, yams and cassava should be limited. Those who are on the Paleo diet have this opinion that if the vegetable cannot be consumed raw, it should be eliminated from the diet.
- **Seeds And Nuts** - Except for peanuts, all nuts and seeds are encouraged. The reason why peanuts are not allowed is because they are legumes. However, you should moderate your consumption as nuts and seeds would probably help you gain weight.

That is if you are on the Paleo diet mainly to lose weight.

- **Meats And Eggs** - Unless you are a vegetarian or vegan, eggs and meats are the main ingredient for the Paleo diet. The thing you need to look out for is to ensure that they are grass-fed products and avoid meats that contain additives and preservatives. Among the best type of meat include beef, chicken, turkey, pork and fish. Among the eggs would include chicken eggs, quail eggs or duck eggs.

- **Oils** - Processed vegetables and hydrogenated oils are heavily discouraged. However, it is recommended to use unprocessed oils such as walnut oil, coconut oil, olive oil and canola oil. Use them in your cooking regularly but at a moderate amount.

- **Beverages To Drink** - Drink a lot of water. Avoid drinking coffee and alcohol. Tea is allowed, provided it doesn't have milk. Fruits and vegetable juices are heavily encouraged.

Among the food you should definitely avoid include:

- **Legumes** - Like said earlier, legumes are not allowed on the Paleo diet. This would include many kinds of beans including kidney beans, black beans, soybeans and mung beans.
- **Grains** - Any cereal grains should be avoided. This would include rice, corn, wheat, oats and barley. Those who have experienced great results from this diet put a lot of emphasis on avoiding white flour and rice as it includes refined carbohydrates.
- **Dairy Products** - Like I said earlier, dairy products are not on the Paleo diet. This includes milk, yogurt, cheese, ice cream and creamer.

Other things to avoid include soft drinks, sweeteners and iodized salt. You should definitely avoid processed foods. Stick to the right food and you would see a great difference to your health and your overall way of life.

Chapter 3 - Starting Off The Paleo Diet

The Paleo diet is a very simple diet compared to other forms of diet. Like mentioned in previous chapters, many other forms of diet include calorie counting and exercising profusely. The Paleo diet focuses on eating natural foods, similarly to those of the hunters and gatherers in the past.

The focus of the Paleo diet is on eating fresh meat, nuts and other fresh food as prescribed in the previous chapter. As such, a lot of the focus would be on preparing yourself for the diet. If you fill your home with proper Paleo food, eating well would come naturally.

As you start off with the Paleo diet, you should start by having an open mind. You would have to sit down and decide when to commit to the diet. Reading this book is a great start as it gives you the right knowledge before you start on this diet.

If you want to go gung ho and go full blast with this diet immediately, then you would have to experience an adjustment period which would last for probably two weeks. This is a tough period which tests a person physically, emotionally and mentally.

In the adjustment period, you should start your diet when your life isn't filled with a lot of stressful situation like a major life change. Certain people would have a terrible headache while other people would have to deal with other symptoms such as flu. They might even feel fatigue, powerful cravings or even dizziness.

Mistakes When Starting Out On The Paleo Diet

Before starting off with the Paleo diet, you should be aware of certain mistakes that most people make when starting off with this diet. Many people make such mistakes because of the common misconception of losing weight. This sub-chapter helps to ensure that you don't make the same mistakes and undo many of the good things that you do.

If applied properly, this diet would create amazing results. If not, you would struggle throughout the entire diet process. Among the common mistakes include:

- **Trying To Completely Eliminate Fat** - Most people who try the Paleo diet are looking to lose weight. As such, they try to eliminate fat completely from their diet. They think that fat is evil and this results in them putting on more weight. This happens because you would need some fat in your diet to help you feel fuller. Without eating fat, you would tend to eat more and binge on more food.
- **Eating Less** - This may be something which surprises you, but eating less doesn't necessarily help you lose weight over the long term. It is better to eat in a more controlled manner. You don't lose weight over the long term by eating less but rather eating healthily. Try eating a more controlled meal on a regular basis. Six healthy meals a day is better than three unhealthy meals.

- **Putting Unnecessary Pressure On Their Body** - Many people think that the process of dieting includes putting pressure on their body. We all crave a treat from time to time. Acknowledge that and start eating some of the "bad foods". One great way is to have a cheat day. A cheat day is a day in the week that allows you to eat anything that you like. Don't go from one extreme to the other when it comes to dieting. Remember, moderation is the key.

- **Eating Excessive Nuts** - In the previous chapter, I have stated that eating nuts is alright. However, many people tend to eat excessively on nuts. My recommendation is that although nuts are allowed in the Paleo Diet, you should try to limit the intake as much as possible. Many people (especially men) start to snack on nuts excessively and believe that it's alright. Eating too much nuts would only put on more weight as they contain fat.

Avoid making such mistakes when you are starting on the Paleo diet. As you understand the reasons for them, you would look to control yourself better. As you take the effort, you would realize that you would lose weight faster and also live healthier.

Tips On Starting Off Paleo Successfully

Starting off with the Paleo diet is easy when you understand the workings of the human body. These are great tips that would help you start off Paleo successfully.

- **Read More About This Diet** - This book provides you great information about the Paleo diet. However, there are other important information such as delicious Paleo recipes and knowledge from other Paleo dieters. You can search for such groups by networking with them on social networking sites. There are also valuable resources in this book.
- **Include Paleo Food In Your Everyday Diet** - Planning ahead is absolutely essential if you want to succeed in the Paleo diet. Foods which are high in carbohydrate, fast foods and whole grain foods can be easily bought from

restaurants or vending machines. Paleo food is definitely more difficult to get. What you need to do is to store your kitchen with heaps of Paleo food that it becomes impossible for you to eat otherwise.

- **Learn About The Best Paleo Food** - Eating a Paleo diet which is rich with protein is better than eating a diet filled with carbohydrates if you are looking to lose weight.

- **Stop With The High Carb Intake** - Those people who take a diet rich with carbohydrate would suffer tremendously when they start a Paleo diet. They would suffer from dizziness and tiredness. It may even stimulate a ketosis problem. Ketosis is a situation that leads to a quick breakdown of body fat. This is extremely risky for those women who are expecting or those who suffer from diabetes.

- **Start With A Detox** - To start off a Paleo diet, you should start with a full body detox first (detox.paleodiet101.info). You could perform a simple body cleanse by taking water with lemon juice, maple syrup and cayenne pepper for a week. Check with your doctor before starting this detox.

- **Start With A Gradual Transition** - Don't start off the Paleo diet immediately. It is better to go slow on the diet. Start to slowly eliminate unhealthy food from your diet and include healthier alternative. This may take up to a month or two. However, you should start to eliminate processed food immediately. You would learn more about this gradual transition in the next sub-chapter.

Dealing With The Transition Period

It should be clear that the Paleo diet is known as a caveman diet. Very few among us would be eating such a diet. Because of our normal conditioning when it comes to eating, switching to a Paleo diet would be very difficult. The elimination of processed foods and agricultural products can be tough considering most of the supermarket is filled with many of these products.

It is normal for those who start out with this Paleo diet to feel a little sluggish in the first few weeks. These are among the tips that you would learn when it comes to dealing with the transitional period.

- **Start Slow** - Nothing is more important than this first tip. It is not easy to transition when it comes to any habits whatsoever. As your body is slowly transitioning to using fat as a form of energy source rather than carbohydrates, you would start to feel slightly shaken and low in energy.

  Don't worry if you have to deal with such symptoms and it is simply a way the body adjusts to a low carbohydrate level. If you feel the dizziness too hard to endure, start by cutting it down slowly. Start with a Paleo meal then slowly build your way to all your meals throughout the day. Then you can slowly reduce the other grains and carbohydrates.

- **Expect A Three Week Adaptation Period** - This is a period where your body would slowly become accustomed to using fat as a source of your daily energy. However, such symptoms would slowly disappear and you will feel that your energy levels would improve.

- **Have Adequate Rest** - Try to sleep as much as you can. Rest is important when you are starting out because you would be low on energy during this period. You should also need to remove stresses in your life as they tend to drain a lot of energy.
- **Exercise Moderately** - You should look to exercise for short bursts rather than long workouts. This is just to ensure that your body gets working. You also need to take extra rest days after exercising.
- **Consult Your Doctor** - Before starting off this diet, you would have to ask your doctor for advice. See if your body is suitable for such a period. Most doctors would be alright with you following this diet. However, the adaptation period might be very turbulent.

Chapter 4 - Cooking For Paleo

Shopping For Paleo

Don't think that shopping for Paleo is a hard thing. Many people believe that just because they are eating a certain diet, they would need to spend a lot of money on buying food. Should you be on a budget, there is a simple method to ensure you get the healthiest food for your money.

A general rule is to always prioritize animal proteins, followed by vegetables, fruits and finally fats. If you are on a budget, you need to spend a bulk of your budget on buying animal protein (meat). Always try to go for organic grass-fed or pasteurized meat.

Look for foods which are fresh. If they are not, go for those on a special to ensure it is worth your money. If you are looking to make lamb for the night but find that there is a special for beef for that day, simply buy the beef and change your recipe. Don't be overly rigid with your recipes.

If you really can't buy certain food because your budget is too tight to afford good quality, you should look to stick to meat from ruminants. This includes goat, venison and lamb. This type of meat has a higher ratio of Omega-3 to Omega-6 compared to other meat like chicken and pork. Buy the leanest cuts and then trim the fat from them. The unhealthy stuff such as toxins, antibiotics and hormones lie within the fat. When it comes to non-organic chicken, you should always eat it without the skin. When it comes to pork, you should try to skip it altogether, unless you can find organic type.

Perhaps my favorite type of animal protein is from fish. As fish is a type of food that couldn't last long, try to cut down on fish if you are on a budget. If you really want to eat it, buy for one meal only unless you plan to freeze it. Less expensive fish would be fishes like scallops or cod.

The most important part of eating a budget Paleo diet is stocking up on eggs. However, there is an important rule here; which is to always buy organic eggs. They are generally more expensive compared to other type of eggs, but they are still a cheaper source of protein compared to other types of meat.

After you have sorted out your animal protein, the next thing to consider is fruits and vegetables. However, you don't have to buy organic. My general recommendation is to spend less on fruits and vegetables and more on better quality meat. Generally, look to buy in season and what's on special. This helps to save you a great deal of money. You should always look to buy your vegetables before you purchase fruit. This is because fruits aren't really necessary. Only buy fruits if your budget permits.

When looking for vegetables, buy leafy and dark vegetables because they have more nutrients. Try to stay away from vegetables such as lettuce, cucumbers and celery since they don't have much nutrition. If you want to save more money, one great way is to purchase frozen vegetables.

After sorting out your animal protein, fruits and vegetables; the next thing is to buy your fats food. Food such as nuts and seeds are great and considered as dietary food. However, be careful of your intake. Try to reduce on them because they can be very expensive. One affordable source of fat includes coconut milk and avocados. Another great way is to preserve olives in salt and water. These are great staples for fats so you should go for them first. Only look to buy nuts and seeds when your budget permits.

When your budget allows you to buy higher priced items such as unrefined coconut oil, extra-virgin olive oil and organic pastured butter; then only do so. They are all great items of fat and would last you for a few months. Herbs and spices are the last thing to consider when buying for a Paleo diet. This would make your daily meals tastier. Adding them to your chicken or beef meal in your meals would make it more interesting. This includes cardamom, cinnamon, cumin and nutmeg.

Always look to purchase the main items first. Don't buy the fruits, nuts and seeds first as they aren't really necessary. Look to buy the main items according to this order: animal protein, vegetables and then fats.

Great Ingredients For Cooking Paleo

It has been clearly mentioned what are the food which you should eat. The allowed meats include any lean beef or pork, poultry and game meat. It is highly encouraged to eat up to six weekly servings of such meat. Fish and shellfish also fall under this category. You should also know that all fruits and non-starch vegetables are allowed. You should try to snack on nuts and seeds. These include almonds, sunflower seeds and pumpkin seeds.

However, you don't have to be completely strict about the Paleo diet. You still can have some food on a moderate basis. This includes olive, canola and other types of oils. However, they shouldn't exceed 4 teaspoons. This is the same for diet sodas, coffee and tea. Other beverages such as wine, beer or spirits should also be limited.

Regardless, there are still many foods which are completely prohibited. The main one is dairy products. Also look to avoid fatty meals, processed foods and starchy vegetables. Although the Paleo diet might seem like a strict diet, there should be some 'cheat days' where you eat what you like. However, you should always learn to control yourself. Don't go overboard with the eating until you lose weight.

Tomatoes In The Paleo Diet

When adapting to the Paleo diet, tomatoes are one of the recommended food under the Paleo diet. It serves as a great anticancer agent and you should adapt to your Paleo diet as closely as possible. From here, you would learn the various ways where you can use tomatoes in your diet.

- **Eat It Raw** - Tomatoes are great to eat raw as it will preserve the nutrients which it has to offer. Its soft texture is also great to put on burgers or sandwiches. If you like, you can also make fresh salads with it. I love it when I mix them with some lettuce, red onion, and avocado with some lemon juice as dressing.
- **Gazpacho** - Gazpacho is a type of cold soup which is filled with vegetables and made of tomato broth base. Tomatoes are without a

doubt, the main ingredient. Other vegetables and herbs are blended together in a food processor. This Gazpacho is a raw recipe which doesn't require additional cooking or heating.

- **Spicy Tomato Soup** - Use eight fresh tomatoes and puree them. Cook a variety of different vegetables plus seasonings to create the spicy tomato soup. It would taste better with some chicken broth. If you are a vegetarian, simply substitute it with vegetable broth.

- **Baked Tomatoes** - The great thing about baked tomatoes is that you the soft fleshy texture is still maintained while adding some heat and roasted flavor. Tomatoes can be combined with other vegetables which you intend to bake in the oven. Try adding some asparagus and eggplant and they would go well with it. Bake them together with some chopped garlic, black pepper and a sprinkle of parsley.

Paleo Tools For Cooking

When it comes to eating a Paleo diet, it requires a great change of the dietary habits as well as general food preference. The most Paleo-friendly foods are raw food. As such, you should make sure that you have tools for making such food such as smoothies and salads.

To make great salad, an attractive set of wooden salad bowls and a cutting board for cutting fresh vegetables. You should also have get a high quality blender such as the Blendtec.

The **Blendtec blender** is a tool that you should definitely get. It has helped me create many Paleo foods easily. You would be able to make plenty of food easily. It is amazing how the blender is able to obtain every single bit of the food that you blend.

Check out the product at

blendtec.paleodiet101.info

As said in previous chapters, meat and protein is an incredibly important ingredient for the Paleo diet. You should look to get a good roasting pan or griddle. Such products help to ensure that the meat wouldn't get stick to the surface of the person's appliances. This would make them want to stick to their dietary goals and give them a better excuse to cook more.

Paleo Cooking Skills

When it comes to cooking Paleo food, it doesn't have to be something difficult. The transitional period may be slightly difficult, but as you develop the right cooking skills, you could learn to cook excellent recipes easily.

This book doesn't go into detail on the different ways of cooking which can save you both money and time. However, I have included another valuable guide where you could purchase. This is a guide which has helped me kick start my Paleo diet in the past.

In This Guide, You Would Learn How To:

- *Cook Quick And Easy Meals That Taste Fantastic*
- *Create Endless Food Choices*
- *Avoid 'Paleo Boredom'*

- *Save On Your Food Bill By Using Ingredient Efficiently*
- *Have A BANK Of Recipes Under Your Belt*

In this guide, you would also have a great bunch of recipes which include:-

- Paleo Smoothie Recipes
- Paleo Dessert Recipes
- Paleo Breakfast Recipes
- Paleo Dinner Recipes
- Paleo FOD Box Recipes
- 1-Click FOD Box Builder
- 1-Click Smoothie Builder

To find out more about this great guide, check out:-

paleoinakitchen.paleodiet101.info

Chapter 5 - Great Paleo Recipes

In this chapter, you would learn a few basic recipes that could help you get started with the Paleo Diet.

However, if you find that this recipe is insufficient, you can check out:-

cookbook.paleodiet101.info

The **Paleo Cookbook** has a great collection of recipes that would help you start your recipe easily…

From this link, you would get a FREE book titled **'Herbs and Spices Using Seasonings in a Paleo Friendly Kitchen'**. This is a great guide which could be incredibly helpful for someone wanting to start the Paleo cooking habit.

Easy Salad With Eggs For Breakfast

Ingredients

- 4 Organic Eggs
- 2 Tablespoons Of Grass-Fed Butter
- 4 Cups Of Mixture Of Spinach And Arugula
- Mixture 1
  - 1/4 Onion, Chopped
  - 1 Persian Cucumber, Sliced
  - 1/2 Green Pepper, Chopped
  - 1 Tomato, Chopped
  - 1 Avocado, Cubed
- Mixture 2 (A Small Dash Each)
  - Organic Dried Dill Weed
  - Dried Oregano
  - Sea Salt
  - Coarse Group Black Pepper
- Extra Virgin Olive Oil

Steps

1. Melt the grass-fed butter over medium heat on a small frying pan.
2. Crack 2 eggs into the pan.
3. Once the butter is melted, cover the pan with a lid.
4. Wash and split the spinach and arugula. Split them on two plates that you would serve on.
5. Top it with Mixture 1.
6. Cook the eggs until a desired consistency.
7. Season it with mixture 2.
8. Drizzle it with the olive oil.
9. Top each plate of salad with 2 cooked eggs.
10. Serve

Tasty Pork Sausage and Onions

Ingredients

- 1 Pound Of Pork Sausage
- Mixture 1
  - 1 Large Onion, Peel And Sliced
  - 2 Bell Peppers, Sliced
  - 1 Apple, Core And Sliced
  - 2 Jalapenos - Remove The Seeds And Sliced
- Mixture 2
  - 3 Tablespoons Of Olive Oil, Melted
  - 1 Lemon, Juiced
- Dried Thyme, To Taste
- Salt And Pepper, To Taste

Steps

1. Preheat the oven to 190 Celsius.
2. Insert Mixture 1 in a 12-inch cast iron skillet.

3. Add Mixture 2 and mix well, ensure an even coating.
4. Sprinkle with Salt and Pepper to the taste of your liking.
5. Take the sausages and place them on the bed of vegetables.
6. Poke 10 holes using a sharp knife around each sausage. This is to ensure they won't explode in the oven.
7. Cover your pan or dish with an aluminum foil and place in the preheated oven.
8. Remove the aluminum foil after 25 minutes. This is to allow the sausages to brown until finished.
9. Remove from the oven once done and sprinkle with dried thyme.
10. Ready to serve.

Roast Bacon Omelet With Sweet Potato

This is a post-workout dish as it is high in carbohydrates. It could be used for a dinner or lunch meal as well. Try to roast the sweet potato the night before. You could also store some of them for an omelet for the very next day. This serves around 2 servings.

Ingredients

Sweet Potato Mixture

- Mixture 1:
  - 1 1/2 Cup Of Diced Sweet Potato
  - 1 Small White Onion, Cut It In Half And Sliced Roughly
  - Few Springs Of Fresh Thyme
- A Pinch Of Sea Salt
- 1 Tablespoon Coconut Oil

Other Mixture

- 6 Whisked Eggs
- A Pinch Of Black Pepper
- 3-4 Rashes Of Bacon
- Ghee Or Coconut Oil, A Dash
- Crumbled Goat's Cheese
- Mixed Salad Greens & Sliced Cucumber

Steps

1. Pre-heat the oven to 200 Celsius.
2. Rub the baking tray with some coconut oil. Let it melt in the oven.
3. Scatter Mixture 1 in a tray and roast in the oven for 30 minutes. Stir it a few times after 15 minutes of roasting. Sprinkle some salt.
4. Remove the rind of the bacon but don't throw it away. Dice the bacon including the fat in the streaky rushes, into small cubes.
5. Cut the rind strips to 4 pieces. Heat a little ghee or coconut oil in a frying pan you would cook the omelet in.

6. Fry bacon for around 5 minutes. Stir frequently until it is brown and crispy. Turn the heat to medium.

7. Add sweet potato mixture and stir until it is warmed up.

8. Pour the whisked egg mixture over the potato and bacon. Ensure the whole surface is covered evenly. Cook for around 5 minutes or until the egg is done. Cover the pan with a lid to speed up the process. Scatter some goat's cheese and black pepper halfway through.

9. Serve with a side salad. This could be a mixture of cucumber, greens, lemon juice and olive oil.

The Basic Burger For Paleos

Ingredients

- 1 Pound Of Ground Beef
- Mixture 1:
  - 10 Sundried Tomatoes, Diced
  - 1/2 Container Of Mushrooms, Diced
- 1/2 Red Onion, Diced
- 2 Tablespoons Of Apple Cider Vinegar
- 1 Tablespoon Of Garlic Power
- 1 Tablespoon Of Onion Powder
- 2 Tablespoon Of Duck Fat
- Salt And Pepper, To Taste

Steps

1. Heat up a skillet with the duck fat.
2. Insert the diced onions into the skillet. Let them cook for a while.
3. Insert Mixture 1 into the skillet.
4. Add apple cider vinegar to the skillet. Let them cook.

5. While they are mixing together, take out the ground beef and make ball-sized balls of meat. Flatten them with your hand to form a burger patty.

6. Add some salt and pepper to your skillet mixture. Once the onions and mushrooms are cooked down, simply add a spoonful of the mixture to the patty and top another patty over that patty.

7. Close the patties up by pinching the sides until they are tightly sealed. Sprinkle the tops of the patties with some garlic and onion powder. This would make it smell very nice.

8. Once the burgers are sealed up, heat up another large skillet with 2 tablespoon of fat.

9. Add the burgers to the pan and let it cook on both sides. This should be around 5 minutes for each side.

10. Once they are cooked, it is ready to serve.

You can serve them with some bread burgers or simply to eat. Either way, they are incredibly tasty.

Easy-Bake Carrot French Fries

Ingredients

- 8 Large Carrots
- 3 Tablespoons Of Olive Oil
- 1 Teaspoon Of Celtic Sea Salt

Steps

1. Cut the carrots to around 2-inch sections. This is similar like French fries. Recut them to thinner sticks.
2. Toss the carrot sticks with the salt and olive oil.
3. Spread the carrot sticks on a parchment paper baking sheet.
4. Bake at 400° Celsius for 20 minutes. Make sure that the carrots are brown.

Trail Mix For The Lazy Paleo

Ingredients

- 1/2 Cup Of Whole Almonds
- 1/2 Cup Of Raw Pumpkin Seeds
- 1/2 Cup Of Raw Sunflower Seeds
- 1/2 Cup Of Whole Cashews
- 1/2 Cup Of Raisins
- 1/2 Cup Of Dried Blueberries

Steps

1. Simply mix everything together and store in an air-tight container.
2. No cooking required.
3. This makes around 3 cups.
4. You can include any other nuts, seeds or dried fruits.

Beware not to always eat this. Nut can be extremely fattening if taken excessively.

Braised Green Beans With Tomatoes And Onions

Ingredients

- Mixture 1
  - 1 Pound Of Green Beans, Trimmed into 2-inch pieces
  - 14-ounce can of Fire-Roasted Tomatoes, Diced and Drained
  - 3 Cloves Of Garlic, Minced
  - 1 1/2 Cups of Low Sodium Chicken Broth
- 2 Tablespoons Of Butter
- 1 Large Onion, Sliced Thinly
- Freshly Ground Pepper and Kosher Salt

Steps

1. Melt the butter in the large skillet over medium heat.
2. The moment it melts and the foam subsides, throw in the onion, pepper and salt.

3. Add Mixture 1 to cover everything. Increase the heat to high until it comes to boil.
4. Cover the skillet with a lid; reduce the heat to low to produce a constant light simmer.
5. Let the beans simmer for 10 minutes to ensure it is tender. Remove the lid and simmer to reduce the liquid for around 2-3 minutes.
6. Ready to serve.

Easy-Roasted Bacon & Broccoli

Ingredients

- Mixture 1:
  - 2 Bunches Of Broccoli, Cleaned and Cut
  - 5 Cloves Of Garlic, Peeled
  - 4 Slices Of Bacon, Bite-size pieces
- Mixture 2:
  - Macadamia Nut Oil
  - Melted Ghee
  - Melted lard
  - Avocado Oil
  - Salt And Pepper, to taste

Steps

1. Toss Mixture 1 into a gallon-sized Ziploc bag. Store them into a fridge until you are ready to roast them.
2. Preheat the oven to 4ooF when you are ready to roast them.

3. Add some fat in the Ziploc bag together with some salt and freshly ground black pepper.
4. Seal the bag and shake it vigorously.
5. Dump the contents together with Mixture 2 on a foil-lined baking tray.
6. Ensure that it all fits into one layer or the broccoli won't cook properly. It is advisable to oven-roast the broccoli for around 30 minutes; rotate the tray and flipping the content every 10 minutes.
7. Ready to serve. Serve with a squeeze of lemon.

Chicken Almond Salad Asian-Style

Ingredients (3 People)

For salad:

- 3 Cups Of Shredded Cooked Chicken
- 3 Carrots, Peeled And Julienned
- 8 Small Kohlrabi Roots, Peeled And Sliced
- Handful Of Cilantro, Chopped
- Handful Of Basil, Chiffonade Cut
- Large Head Of Romaine Lettuce, Torn Into Bite-Size Pieces

For sauce:

- 2 Tablespoons Fish Sauce
- 3 Tablespoons Creamy Almond Butter
- 2 Tablespoons Of Lime Juice, Freshly Squeeze
- 2 Tablespoons Of Unsweetened Applesauce
- 1 Tablespoon Of Coconut Vinegar
- 1/2 Teaspoon Of Crushed Red Pepper

Steps

1. Combine sauce mixture. Whisk them.
2. Slice the kohlrabi and shred with the carrots with a julienne peeler.
3. Toss it to a bowl and add the dressing, chicken and herbs. Toss them well.
4. Serve on the romaine lettuce.

Cheesy Egg Muffins

Ingredients (6 Muffins)

- Mixture 1
  - 4 large eggs
  - 2 tablespoons of full fat Greek yogurt
  - A Dash of Salt
- Mixture 2
  - 3 tablespoons coconut flour
  - 1/4 teaspoon baking powder
- 1/2 cup of shredded Cheddar cheese
- Kosher salt
- Freshly ground black pepper

Steps

1. Preheat the oven to 375F
2. Insert Mixture 1 into a bowl and whisk it till it blended.
3. Add Mixture 2 and mix the batter till it is smooth.

4. Put in the cheese and some freshly-ground black pepper and stir them together.
5. Insert into a paper cupcake liner that is painted with melted coconut oil.
6. Pop the tray in the oven for around 20 minutes. Rotate the tray halfway during the cooking time.
7. Take the muffins out and let them cool on a rack for around 10 minutes.
8. Serve.

Easy Paleo Frittata

Ingredients

- 1 Cup Of Protein (Any meat you desire)
- 1 Tablespoon Coconut Oil
- 1 Cup Frozen Broccoli
- 4 Eggs
- Mixture 1:
  - 1 Teaspoon Kosher Salt
  - 2 Tablespoons Coconut Milk
  - Freshly-ground Black Pepper

Steps

1. Preheat the toaster oven to 350 Celsius.
2. Heat the coconut oil in an 8-inch cast iron skillet over medium heat.
3. Add the cup of protein (meat) to the skillet and stir-fry until heated.
4. Place the frozen broccoli in a microwave-safe bowl. Cover it with a wet paper towel, nuke it till it's thawed.

5. Cut the broccoli into bite-sized pieces with a knife.
6. Add broccoli to ingredients in the pan and mix until cook thoroughly.
7. Crack eggs into a bowl and add Mixture 1.
8. Pour egg mixture into skillet and cook for a few minutes or until the bottom of the frittata is ready.
9. Place skillet into oven.
10. Cook for 15 minutes. Increase the heat to boil for another 2 minutes or until it is puffs up and cooked all the way through.
11. Take it out and transfer the frittata to a plate, sliced.
12. Serve.

5 Minute Paleo Crab Salad

Ingredients (3 People)

- 1 Pound Of Can Lump Crab Meat
- Mixture 1:
  - 2 Scallions, Thinly Sliced
  - 2 Tablespoons Of Chopped Italian Parsley
  - Freshly-ground Black Pepper
  - Kosher Salt
- Mixture 2:
  - 1 Tablespoon Of Lemon Juice
  - 2 Tablespoons Of Paleo Mayonnaise

Steps

1. Open the can of lump crab meat. Squeeze out the extra liquid. Dumb the crab in a bowl.
2. Insert Mixture 1.
3. Add Mixture 2.
4. Taste to see if you would need extra lemon juice, salt, pepper or mayonnaise.
5. Serve over some green. You can top it with some avocado.

Sausage Egg Mcmuffin Paleo

Ingredients

- 2 Large Eggs
- Kosher Salt
- Freshly-ground Black Pepper
- 1/4 Cup Of Water
- 1 Heaping Tablespoon Guacamole
- 2 Tablespoons Of Ghee, Divided
- 1/4 Pound Bulk Raw Pork Sausage

Steps

1. Grease two stainless steel 3.5-inch biscuit cutters on the inside with melted ghee.
2. Place a cutter on a plate and fill it with the sausage meat.
3. Press the meat down gently to shape a sausage patty.
4. Heat a skillet over medium heat and add a tablespoon of ghee.

5. Add patty to the pan when the fat is shimmering.
6. Keep the mold on to ensure that they are shaped properly.
7. Clean the biscuit cutter and grease it again.
8. Fry the sausage for around 3 minutes on each side until fully cooked.
9. Grab two small bowls and crack an egg into each. Pierce the yolks with a fork.
10. Heat a skillet over medium-high heat with the remaining tablespoon of ghee.
11. Once the ghee shimmers, place the two greased biscuit cutters in the pan and pour an egg into each mold. Season it with some salt and pepper.
12. Add 1/4 cup of water to the skillet. Ensure not to splash the eggs. Turn the heat to low and cover the pan.
13. Cook the eggs for around 2 minutes or until it is cooked.
14. Transfer the eggs to a paper-towel lined plate.
15. Sandwiching the sausage (McMuffin) between two egg rounds.
16. Serve.

Chapter 6 - Exercising When On The Paleo Diet

Losing weight is something anybody could do irrespective of sex or age. With a simple and light workout of three times a day, you would be able to lose your chubbiness in no time at all. You could quicken the process by eating right as well.

Exercising isn't even necessary if you eat right. The Paleo diet is highly effective in allowing your body to obtain enough nutrition from food to help you gain fitness from exercising and lose weight fast.

The Paleo diet is also effective in helping you build up lean muscles. You would be able to get your dream body provided you aren't looking for a bulky muscular body. Proper eating combined with light, consistent workout could help create a lean body. You don't have to work out intensely to lose weight. However, if you are keen to obtain extra fitness or muscle mass, you should consider hiring a personal trainer.

The people who work out heavily are those who normally want to build bulky muscles. However, this cannot happen as this diet is natural and doesn't cause an artificial building of muscle. Most muscle building programs now are essentially artificial building of the muscle by taking processed supplements. However, you could still gain healthy lean muscles with the Paleo diet.

Focus On Heart And Lungs

For those who are on the Paleo diet, try to focus your exercise more on cardio exercises. Cardio exercises are great to improve the function of the heart. This would make you stronger and also help you reduce weight.

Cardio exercises include exercises such as walking, running or swimming. The best exercise for staying fit naturally is to pick up running. When you run, your heart rate is made to vary.

There is great impact on your whole body as it would help in building up the tissue and strengthening the bones.

Cycling is also another great activity for the heart. Cycling for an hour a day could help you burn around 500 calories and also build some muscle on your lower body. Swimming is another great activity as it helps to improve blood circulation and improves lung capacity.

Apart from such cardio exercises, you could also consider other repetitive workouts. These include weight lifting, sit-ups and push-ups. You can also try some martial arts like kickboxing or karate. However, having a personal guide is important to ensure that you perform them properly and don't injure yourself

If possible, try to get a body massage whenever possible. When your body is being massaged, it becomes very relaxed and lowers the body stress levels. Your body would feel more comfortable and you would even feel more comfortable expressing your feelings.

I have seen people crying uncontrollably after a massage because they have allowed themselves to be vulnerable due to the relaxation. Don't worry as this is a good thing. It is like a 'detox' of your emotions. A good advice is to not eat anything for at least an hour before a massage. This is because with food in your stomach, the body's metabolism couldn't relax and the massage wouldn't be that effective.

Gaining Muscles

Although it has been stated that you cannot build bulky muscles with the Paleo diet, it is still very possible to build some lean muscles if you follow certain guidelines. These are some tips that would help you gain some lean muscles over a four week period.

- **Start Slow Then Train Hard**. If you want to build muscles, you would need to give them some stimulation for them to grow. You must train with weight resistance. Focus on exercises which work out the big muscles. This includes bench presses, deadlifts and squats. Start off slow and then slowly increase the intensity. Also make sure that you don't train too often as your muscle wouldn't be stimulated for muscle growth.

- **Eat Quality Meat**. Good meat may cost more but they are great for building up muscles. Muscles are made of protein and after you trained hard, you would need plenty of them. Try to have it at least three times a day. A basic rule is to consume between one to two grams of protein for each pound of body weight.

- **Have A High Calorie Snack**. Not only is consuming food regularly important, you should also try to eat a high calorie snack to help prevent hunger. The energy you eat would help you build muscle mass easier. Nut and dried fruit mixed together is one of my favorite.

- **Sleep Well**. When you are sleeping, the body recovers. If it doesn't recover, it doesn't grow. Make sure that you have adequate rest daily. Ideally speaking, you should have at least eight hours of good sleep. Try sleeping in a pitch black room to ensure that you could sleep well.

Paleo Diet For Athletes

Athletes are known to try many different diets to help enhance performance. The Paleo diet is a diet that was created by coaches, nutritionists and doctors. It is a healthy diet for athletes. Human beings are programmed genetically to do well on the Paleo diet. This is because the Paleo diet has high protein which helps enhance performance.

When on the Paleo diet for athletes, you need to focus on the consumption of lean meats. Lean meat contains less fat and one great example is chicken breast. Lean red meats would include cuts with less of a marble effect. The marble effect is a situation where the white fat end up mixed with the red meat. This is normally affected in meats like sirloin, top round and T-bone.

Eggs are also a great ingredient for athletes as the protein would help you repair stressed muscles. Eggs are a great ingredient for your breakfast preparation. Try finding for eggs which come from organically raised chickens.

Seafood is also an important aspect of the Paleo diet. It provides lean protein. Salmon also provides omega-3 fatty acids which are good for the joint.

Fruits and vegetables are another major source of the Paleo diet for athletes. You should ensure that vegetables are included in every meal that you eat. However, not all vegetables need to be eaten raw. Fruits are not necessary in fact, but you could take some fruits from time to time.

Athletes who are looking to enhance their performance should look to try the Paleo diet. It is a great diet for athletes and you would look to try it if you are an athlete.

Chapter 7 - Intermittent Feasting

The Paleo Diet, when combined with **Intermittent Feasting**, would be able to get you great weight loss results. Of course, it would also provide you with great health benefits over a period of time.

The Intermittent Feast, or Alternate Day Fasting, involves an alternate day of fasting followed by a day of eating regularly. On your fasting day, you would eat very little and then eat normally (or more) on the very next day. This method is very attractive for many people for obvious reasons.

Knowing that we could indulge in our favorite food the next day may make dieting today more bearable. Scientists have proven that alternate day fasting wouldn't just help us lose weight but also make us healthier over the long term as well. It would reduce other health problems such as cancer, heart disease and ease asthma symptoms too.

This idea of restricting calories came about in the year 2003. A lab research conducted by the National Institute on Aging in America found staggering results when such a method of eating is implemented. Although the research was done on mice, it is substantive to prove that it can help you greatly. They aren't many human studies to prove this theory and a lot of research has to be done in order to draw any substantive conclusions.

Without a doubt, restricting the calories intake would normally result in weight loss. However, using the Intermittent Feasting diet provides greater long term results. Another study conducted was published in the American Journal of Clinical Nutrition proved greatly how this diet can help aid weight loss.

In this study, sixteen normal weight adults follow an alternate day regime of fasting and feasting for three weeks. During the fasting days, they had only calorie-free drinks while they were allowed to eat whatever they wanted on feasting days.

The results showed that by the end of the study, the participant lost an average of 3 percent of their initial body weight and lost four percent of their fat mass. However, it was hard to sustain this eating period for too long because most of the participants would feel extremely hungry during this study.

As such, the scientists behind this study suggested that it would be better if it was allowed a small meal on fasting day. That is the base of the Intermittent diet. The idea is to restrict your calorie intake to just one fifth of what you normally eat.

On the first day of the diet, you restrict the food intake to just one-fifth of the calories you normally take. Generally, women need around 2000 calories a day while men need 2500 calories a day. As such, women would eat 400 calories and men would take 500 calories on this first day. However, this is also dependent on your weight. If you are heavier, you would need more calories.

On the second day of your diet, you would simply eat what you normally eat.

On the third day, you start with the same as day one. Continue from here for a few weeks, preferably a minimum of two weeks.

After a few weeks under this regime, you should be able to lose weight.

However, it has to be noted that the reason why you can lose weight from this diet is more than just because of the reduction of calories intake. Another reason for the weight loss is because fasting every other day would help to activate a form of skinny gene known as SIRT1. This gene helps boost weight loss further and also improve your health.

SIRT1 works in a complicated way. The idea is that when cells are restricted of energy, they would become 'stressed' and the cells would start to die. This activates SIRT1, which would set off a process of stopping the cells from dying.

This gene would also help to make our metabolism more efficient so that you would be able to burn fat better. Besides that, the SIRT1 would also inhibit substances in the bodies which cause inflammation. This is extremely important because inflammation causes many health problems like cancer, heart diseases, asthma and premature aging.

Before you decide to start with this diet, you should always check with your doctor first. This diet may not be suitable for everyone. An example of this is people with diabetes. Eating too little on certain days would not be suitable when they are on regular medication. As such, always check with your doctor.

However, despite all the benefits of Intermittent Feasting, there are also certain things that you would need to consider. You need to guard against bingeing on the 'feast' days. Many people, after fasting for a full day, would end up eating like a mad person. As such, it is still important to control your diet on 'feast' days.

Another big disadvantage of the intermittent feast is if your diet is unhealthy in the very first place, you won't be able to get the benefits. If you continue to eat unhealthy on your 'feast' days, you wouldn't be able to get the results you want. As such, you should try to implement the Paleo diet together with the intermittent feasting. On the 'feast' days, you should have a Paleo diet. Try eating foods which are filled with healthy nutrients on feast days.

Feasting days should consist of plenty of vegetables, fruits and low-fat protein-rich food.

Ultimately, following this intermittent feasting together with the Paleo Diet would help you lose weight and regain your health. You wouldn't feel overly deprived. Other diets would make you feel deprived because you are constantly deprived of your favorite food. This form of dieting allows you to eat normally and not worry too much about eating the low calorie options.

To find out more about the Intermittent Feast, check out:

intermittentfeast.paleodiet101.info

Chapter 8 - Paleo Skincare

The Paleo Diet is a kind of diet which has multiple benefits. However, what haven't been talked about are the possible benefits on your skin as well as other potential health issues. This includes conditions such as acne, eczema, scarring, weak hair and psoriasis. These are all serious conditions that can create a lot of problem for those who have them.

Many of us have been misled and confused when it comes to caring for their skin. Many products simply make you more dependent on them while not providing you with proper benefits to deal with your condition. Many of us go to great lengths to avoid chemicals and man-made ingredients in our food, but what we put on the outside of our body can also affect our skin deeply.

As the Paleo diet doesn't allow the consumption of processed food, you also wouldn't need to put a whole load of chemical cocktails to maintain a great complexion. Simply using natural options is not only less expensive, but also more effective and easier.

At its core, the Paleo diet is a diet which increases the health of your skin because it is a diet filled with rich protein and healthy fats. Skin is comprised of fats and with healthy fats, you would be able to provide your skin with the necessary tools to repair the skin and maintain its elasticity. It is the elasticity of the skin which provides a youthful appearance. Besides that, eating this diet provides great nutrients and vitamins that are important for glowing skin.

The two main foods that sabotage the health of our skin are grains and dairy. The Paleo diet prohibits both those food. If you are someone who eats plenty of grains and diary, it would lead to acne and other sorts of skin problems. There are other great benefits of the Paleo diet.

Among the various nutrients of Paleo food includes:

- **Nuts** - Particularly almond, aren't only a great snack, but contain healthy fats which would improve your skin. It also has high levels of Vitamin E. Vitamin E is a nutrient which moisturizes the skin.
- **Fish** - This is the best source of Omega-3 Fats. They are not only healthy for your heart but they are also great in helping to slow down the aging process and improve skin elasticity. Omega-3 also fights possible inflammation from free radicals in the body, a main reason we develop acne.
- **Chicken** - Chicken is the main source of food on the Paleo diet. It is an important source of protein and it is important for beautiful skin.
- **Eggs** - Another staple of the Paleo diet. They are not only taste but can be cooked easily too. Similarly, they are packed with protein that is the building block of great skin.
- **Tomatoes** - They are full with lycopene, an important ingredient in fighting blemishes. They also contain antioxidants that help ensure that your skin is free from toxins and free radicals. Free radicals are known to speed-up the aging process.

The **<u>Skintervention Guide</u>** is the best guide I have seen in improving your skin, teeth and hair naturally. This guide isn't just for people who suffer from these problems. It is also a valuable guide for those who want healthier skin, stronger teeth and better hair. This guide truly tackles it all. This is a comprehensive guide for self-care, home-care and everything else.

This guide contains:

- More than 200 pages of information that would change the way you think about skincare
- **Two EXTRA Bonus - Skintervention Guide Easy Recipes and Skintervention Guide Resources**
- The nutrients you need for beautiful outlook appearances
- Knowing how to improve your digestive system
- Alternative to conventional makeup
- Tips for smart intimate and feminine care
- How to ditch food toxins in your body

From this guide, you would learn how to have:
- Natural Beautiful Skin

- Radiant And Strong Hair And Nails
- Being Free From Using Commercial Products And Media Brainwashing
- Use The Body To Your Own Advantage
- Knowing How To Choose The Proper Makeup For Your Skin
- The Best Way To Nourish Your Body

Get the guide from

primalskincare.paleodiet101.info

Resource 1 - Paleo 30 Day Challenge

You have learned a great deal about the Paleo diet. Now it's time to put it into practice.

However, finding the discipline to implement it might be easier said than done. Anyone who has tried any new diet would easily attest to this.

The answer to starting out the Paleo diet successfully would be the **Paleo 30 Day Challenge**.

This guide is designed to help you throughout the entire time to maximize your success. This guide includes many things, including:

- A solid foundation of knowledge with regards to the Paleo diet
- A help through the "little challenges" of the resistance period
- Understanding why fat wouldn't necessarily make you fat

- The reason why you should eat more salt
- Why spending time on the treadmill isn't entirely good
- Why it is okay to eat whenever you are hungry
- **A FULL FOUR WEEKS MEAL PLAN**

There are many delicious meals that you can create from this guide, including:

- ✓ *Jambalaya*
- ✓ *Tuna Salad Sandwiches*
- ✓ *Salmon Quiche*
- ✓ *Berry Cobbler Delight*
- ✓ *Breakfast Pizza*
- ✓ *Chicken Fajitas*

...which are all Paleo-based food.

What's more, you even have a **complete grocery list** to help you start off easily too.

In the member's area, you would also have many resources including:

- ➢ **VIP Paleo Cooking Class**
- ➢ **VIP Discount On Beef**
- ➢ **Interviews With Experts On Paleo And Other Nutrition**

It is difficult to start off this diet. As such, a custom-made log is included to track your progress throughout the way.

Not only that, you would also have a free copy of **The Gastronomical Caveman Cookbook**. It is a great guide which includes another 80 special recipes.

Get the Paleo 30 Day Challenge now at

30day.paleodiet101.info

Resource 2 - Fat Loss Factor

If you are someone who is constantly disappointed by diet programs, the **Fat Loss Factor System** is what you need. This system is essential if you want to achieve your dream body over a short period of time.

This guide is special because it contains the methods of having a healthy lifestyle program that would help to lose unwanted belly fat. What makes this guide so effective is because it deals with the mental aspect of losing weight first. From here, you would learn the aspect of eating better, exercising well and creating a focused mental attitude.

A big part of this system includes knowing how to remove bad toxins from your body. You would learn how to eat certain fruits like vegetables, fruits and nuts.

In summary, this program offers the following steps to lose weight naturally:

- The first part is the <u>clean-slate step</u> where the person is allowed to eat natural meals such as fruits, nuts, vegetables and legumes.
- The next part is about <u>proper exercise and eating a balanced diet</u>. This program offers various workout plans from the beginner to an expert.

This system works by <u>combining nutrition, two fat loss techniques, proper workouts and caloric shifting</u>. The process of caloric shifting helps you to focus on eating various amounts of calories at different times and days. This would confuse your body and this forces it to gain metabolism. Increasing your metabolism is a great way to lose weight.

In short, the Fat Loss Factor Program contains these advantages:

- ***You don't have to take harmful substance chemicals to lose weight.***
- *It is easy-to-follow which is suitable for everyone.*

- *You can experience rapid fat loss from the beginning.*
- *You will develop a stronger physique*
- *It is well-organized and makes people follow it effortlessly.*
- *Experience higher energy level*
- *Includes eBooks and videos*
- *Workout plans*
- *Healthy food lists & Recipes*

Check out this amazing program at:

fatloss.paleodiet101.info